HORMONES
HEALTH
AND
YOU

ISBN: 978-1-63308-486-5 (paperback)
　　　 978-1-63308-487-2 (ebook)

Interior Design by *R'tor John D. Maghuyop*

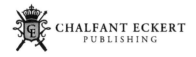

CHALFANT ECKERT
PUBLISHING

1028 S Bishop Avenue, Dept. 178
Rolla, MO 65401

Printed in United States of America

HORMONES
HEALTH
AND
YOU

BIOIDENTICAL
HORMONES
MADE SIMPLE

SUSAN BERKEY

reviewed by
Charles W. Cather R.Ph., M.B.A., FASCP

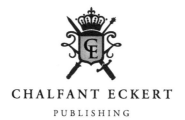

CHALFANT ECKERT
PUBLISHING

I dedicate this book to the one person who was always at the fore front of my mind, as I navigate through my health struggles and forged my own path to healing.

*Mom - you never left my side in spirit,
and I will forever wonder what life could have been for you,
had I known all that I know now.*

TABLE OF CONTENTS

ACKNOWLEDGMENTS

I am the last person that I ever thought would be able to put my passion for research into a published book. However, my determination to help women overcome their health issues and to be proactive with their health became my motivating force.

Many people helped make the completion of this book a reality. First and foremost, I want to thank God for guiding me and giving me the passion for helping women gain the knowledge to live their lives to the fullest and free of disease for many, many years.

I was introduced to the wonderful benefits of alternative care through Dr. Jeffrey Fedorko, D.C., more than 20 years ago. He is a chiropractor/kinesiologist with incredible knowledge of how the body works and what we need to do to stay healthy. I have the utmost admiration for his drive to make a difference. He changed my life.

A person to whom I owe my deepest gratitude is Tom Frye, P.D., a dear friend, as well as a very knowledgeable compounding pharmacist. He opened my eyes and gave me the information I needed to begin my research with bioidentical hormones, which I believe gave me a whole new life.

I also owe a great deal of thanks and gratitude to Dr. William Emley, D.C., for his compassion, care, and guidance. He is a chiropractor/kinesiologist that has given me nutritional guidance and chiropractic care for many years. He is always encouraging me and supporting my passion.

Another inspirational person in my life is my hero, Dr. John R. Lee, M.D., author of *What Your Doctor May Not Tell You About Menopause: The Breakthrough Book on Natural Hormone Balance* (2004). He was a visionary in the field of progesterone, dedicating over 30 years, researching the benefits of progesterone replacement in women. Many of us women will always be grateful for his many years of dedication.

Charles Cather is an extremely knowledgeable compounding pharmacist. He hired me to do marketing for his compounding pharmacy. My job was to introduce doctors to bioidentical hormones and to ensure them that he could fulfill their compounding needs. This was very exciting for me because this has been my passion for many years. I will always be grateful for that opportunity. He has also been kind enough to do hormone consults free of charge for my clients. He has taught me so much over the years. My thanks and gratitude are boundless.

I want to thank my daughter, Lauren, a very creative and dedicated graphic design artist. She is responsible for the beautiful book jacket.

Many thanks to the following people for their knowledge and numerous hours that they gave helping me with the editing process: Kristy Van Camp, Daphne Midcap, Dee Lakes, Kathleen Lapchinski, Cherry Kassebaum, Jared Cavileer, Marie Elana Kennedy, and Dave Prewitt. Without their editing skills, my book would have never made it to completion.

A special thanks to Donna Nowak, a former editor for **Balanced Living** magazine and former CEO of the American Holistic Medical Association, who took the time out of her very busy schedule to help finalize my manuscript for publication. She has an enormous wealth of knowledge in the editing field, and I felt I was very blessed that she offered to give of her time to make my dream a reality. Her comments, suggestions, and support meant the world to me. My gratitude for her contribution is boundless.

Kendra Shea is another special person that provided invaluable assistance. She gave me the motivation to continue the completion of my book – pulling it together, providing the final touches and making sure I came off well and accurately. Her encouragement, creative style, and valuable editing skills were major contributions. I will always be thankful for her help. It took years from start to finish. Without Kendra's patience and guidance, I wouldn't be here today.

AUTHOR'S NOTE

When I first sat down to write this book, my mother was at the forefront of my mind. The memory of her struggles was the driving force behind my desire to inform and educate women on the options that are available to them as they begin to age and experience the dreaded "change of life."

As I approached adulthood, the realization that I was mirroring many of my mother's health issues and diseases was disconcerting. I was determined to do research and make appropriate life changes so that I would not live my mother's life. She suffered from a myriad of illnesses such as adrenal insufficiency, hypothyroidism, fibromyalgia, and severe osteoporosis. She was not always that way. She had a very active life and was an avid swimmer and sports lover; she was even named "Miss Fort Jackson" during World War II. But as she aged, her body began to deteriorate, as well as her quality of life.

Tom Frye, a dear friend, and compounding pharmacist changed my life by introducing me to bioidentical hormones. After experiencing hormonal changes in my late 40s, he suggested I use progesterone to combat my symptoms. As my symptoms abated, my curiosity grew, and my search for the answers to understanding my body and overall health intensified.

The experience of writing this book has been a labor of love, and there have been times where I have had to set my work aside due to the unpredictability of life. When I look back now, I am grateful for life's little interruptions because my purpose for writing this book has evolved into something greater than the clichéd fear of "becoming my mother." My children entered adulthood. They became wives and mothers. The importance of sustaining the health of my family and their families eventually became the driving force behind this book.

Although the priorities of my research have expanded and deepened far beyond bioidentical hormones, the foundation for overall health for women starts with understanding what makes us unique, and hormonal balance plays an important part of that journey. I have witnessed, firsthand, the health benefits that can be attained simply by arming yourself with knowledge. Understanding your body and having the knowledge to ask informed questions of your health care providers can lead to empowering solutions that will improve your quality of life. If this book assists just one woman on her journey to overall wellness, I will judge this personal mission as a success.

—Susan Berkey

FOREWORDS

Susan's natural curiosity and dedication to understand her own medical struggles has created her genuine desire to assist other women on their journey to a proactive approach to hormones and their health. She has an innate ability to take complex medical information and help the average woman make informed decisions regarding hormone health.

Susan worked with me for two years marketing the option of compounding bioidentical hormones. She visited many doctors and addressed the importance of hormone balance with the option of using bioidentical pharmaceuticals. Because of the knowledge she has, she is able to exchange information about BHRT to doctors and create a more open and amiable discussion.

This quick read on bioidentical hormones and treatment options can be used as a guide for professionals as well as patients; empowering all with knowledge that brings value to an important conversation about women's health.

—Charles W. Cather, RPh, MBA, FASCP
Green, OH

This little book offers you two big gifts: a complicated problem made simple and a handy little reference for many answered questions. As a book, it is a short read. As a reference guide, it is full of information that generates an understanding of hormone systems and allows the reader to become more aware of current treatment options for hormone imbalances.

I have known Susan for many years, and as a patient, she has always been inquisitive and wanting to know more. She is fully engaged in her personal health care, being proactive, and taking responsibility for her choices. She reads books from experts in the field, attends numerous seminars, and is always on the lookout for innovative research. She delights in her newfound information and finds it rewarding to help women with their health care. At times, she discloses how her clients find it difficult to understand their own personal health conditions and when they approach their doctors with questions the doctors are either uninformed, misinformed, have no opinion, or beg them off with no time to answer questions. Finding incomplete resources available for women with hormone concerns, Susan set out to create a usable, easy read to empower, inspire, and inform women. I believe she has been quite successful in this regard. If you have concerning hormone issues and are finding it difficult to get answers, this book is for you.

—Jeffrey S. Fedorko, DC
Canton, OH

Susan came to me as a patient in 2012, in search of treatment for adrenal issues and bioidentical hormone therapy. She has always been inquisitive and thirsty for natural approaches to treat her ailments. Her inexhaustible determination to understand her body and achieve optimal health has driven her to dedicate many years to researching the benefits of bioidentical hormones. Bioidentical Hormone Therapy can be an overwhelming topic for the average, everyday woman to digest. Susan navigated the difficult journey to understanding, diagnosing, and treating hormonal issues by arming herself with knowledge and research. Moving forward, she has made it her mission to educate and empower other women, like herself, who are interested in understanding bioidentical hormones and exploring the treatment options that are available to them. This book can serve as a helpful and informational tool for women who are on that same journey and guide them on the path to being proactive participants in their own healthcare.

—Dr. Nancy Fazekus Grubb, M.D., ABFM, ABIHM
Green, OH

Unless faced with a traumatic health situation or potentially fatal diagnosis, most of us don't have the time, inclination, or discipline to study a multitude of books on a particular health topic. Since menopause isn't considered a medical illness anyway, most women have just endured it, asked friends for suggestions, or turned to their family doctor for help. Unfortunately, the result has been a lot of needless suffering. Good for you for finding this little book.

Although the "change of life" may be a natural biological process, it is a complex transition that can wreak havoc on a woman's life. For a lucky few, it's a non-event, an almost transparent transition. For others, symptoms such as depression, hot flashes, sleeplessness, and more become almost unbearable. I had my first hot flash at age 40 with virtually no other symptoms. My body decided to take its good old time, with menopause holding off until age 59. Like many of you reading this book, the final few years were quite a challenge for me with a wide range of troubling symptoms.

For a variety of reasons, taking pharmaceuticals long-term was simply not an option for me, but it was clear that something had to be done. Thanks to my involvement in the holistic community, I was aware of bioidentical hormones and had heard both anecdotal stories and seen limited research about the effectiveness of BHRT. But frankly, my busy lifestyle made it very unlikely that I'd ever delve deeply into the research myself. Susan Berkey kindly served as a helpful sounding board for me on a number of occasions.

Based upon conversations with other women taking bioidentical hormones and information shared by doctors specializing in bioidentical hormone replacement therapy (BHRT), my understanding is that it can take a year or longer to find the combination of hormones that will create balance within each of us. There can be frustration and confusion along the way. In addition, since most insurance companies don't yet cover BHRT, there's a potentially significant out-of-pocket financial investment required to achieve a true state of well-being.

What worked for your best friend, colleague, or neighbor probably won't necessarily work for you. You need a doctor who is knowledgeable in BHRT—one who is wise, patient, and compassionate, and you'll need to have patience, persistence, and discipline yourself. Susan's book can help demystify the process of achieving optimal health through hormonal balance. She is zealous in her study of the subject and generous of heart in sharing what she has learned.

—Donna Nowak, CH, CRT
Cleveland Heights, OH

Susan did a great job at presenting in a concise way the topic of bioidentical hormones. The overview that she presents makes what may seem an impossible subject logical and understandable. I applaud her efforts. Bioidentical Hormone Replacement Therapy is common sense medicine, based on medical research and more than four decades of positive clinical experience. Susan widens the opportunity for more people to be informed and to take advantage of this health restoring approach.

—Joel Yaffa, M.D.
Hainesport, NJ

A great book simplifying the complex world of functional endocrinology, in particular, bioidentical hormones: This book will undoubtedly bridge the communication gap between physician and patient and ultimately empower patients in learning how to best treat their endocrine disorders.

—Dr. William W. Emley, Jr., DC
Bolivar, OH

Susan's book is a wonderful synoptic guide to looking at signs and symptoms of hormone deficiencies and how to evaluate them. I do believe that this guide would be a benefit to anyone who may be having symptoms relating to hormones and to practitioners who need a quick reference.

—Ian Suzelis, DO
Alliance, OH

CHAPTER 1

SYNTHETIC HORMONES VERSUS BIOIDENTICAL HORMONES

"I believe that you are more than your body… that your mind, body, and spirit are inextricably one, inseparable. If you are to achieve lasting vital health, all aspects of your being need to be cared for and loved."
—Dr. Laux, N.D.

Hormones are our own fountain of youth. They assist in regulating almost every function of our body, from our thought processes to the electrical signals in our heart. No longer must we accept the deterioration (both physical and mental) that comes with age. We now know that the quality and length of our lives can be improved by proper hormone balance. I intend to inform women with a description of various hormones so that they may understand how they all work in harmony.

SYNTHETIC HORMONES

It is important to know that bioidentical hormones are not the same as synthetic hormones. In the 1960s, doctors began prescribing an estrogen drug called Premarin®. This synthetic hormone was purported to save women from the horrible symptoms of menopause. Premarin® is manufactured from horse urine—the name stands for pregnant mare's urine—and has been proclaimed as a "natural" substance. It may be natural to horses, but it contains estrogens that are totally foreign to a woman's body. Natural means the exact chemical duplication of what each of us produces in our own body. If women would take a few minutes to research the cruelty shown to mares to produce Premarin® for the sole purpose of financial gain, they might think twice about using it for that reason alone.

Progestin (Provera®) was added to Premarin® in the 1970s because of the risk of endometrial cancer for estrogen users. This new combination is called Prempro®. Adding progestin to estrogen did protect the uterus from developing endometrial cancer, but progestin was found to cause harm as well. Progestin cannot help the body produce or balance hormones. It actually stops the function of progesterone. Many doctors proclaim that Progestin and progesterone are chemically made the same. Progestin is synthetically made by adding chemicals that are not natural in nature. Progesterone, on the other hand, is made identical to the naturally occurring hormone in a woman's body. In 1993, a study called "Women's Health Initiative (WHI)" examined the effects of Premarin® and Prempro®. Unfortunately, the study was discontinued before the completion date of 2005 because of the following findings that were published in JAMA (The Journal of the American Medical Association)

- Breast cancer increased by 26%
- Strokes increased by 41%
- Doubling of rates of venous thromboembolism (blood clots)
- Cardiovascular disease increased by 22%
- Abnormal mammograms increased (35% vs. 23%)
- Breast biopsies increased (10% vs. 6.1%)
- Breast cancer risk increased after one year of use, and the cancers were more advanced when diagnosed
- Dementia or senility was more prevalent in women over 65 using Premarin® and Provera®
- A woman's quality of life did not improve

In this study, which was published in the premier British Medical Journal, *The Lancet* on August 9, 2003, researchers found that a million postmenopausal women who were current users of HRT had a 66% higher risk of developing breast cancer and a 22% higher risk of dying of breast cancer than woman who had never used Premarin® and Prempro®.

In 2001, a government scientific advisory panel voted to add synthetic estrogen to the nation's list of carcinogenic agents.

"Synthetic hormones are made by altering the molecular structure of a hormone enough so that it can be patented. These maintain some of the activity of the natural hormone, but any change in the three-dimensional structure of a hormone, no matter how small, changes its biological effects on the cell in ways that are not completely understood. Frankly, I trust the wisdom coming from Mother Nature's millions of years of experimentation much more than I trust fifty years of biochemical wizardry from Father Pharmaceutical."

Christiane Northrup, M.D., author of *The Wisdom of Menopause,* 2006, revised 2012.

BIOIDENTICAL HORMONES

Twenty years ago, pioneering doctors and health care professionals listened to numerous complaints from women about side effects of hormone replacement therapy (HRT). They began working to provide an alternative to Premarin® and Provera® that would not have the negative side effects or long-term health risks. Unlike synthetic hormones, bioidentical hormones are a perfect match to the hormones a woman's body naturally produces. They are considered identical to the naturally occurring human hormones because they duplicate the molecular structure of our intricate endocrine system exactly. Bioidentical hormones have been used in Europe for 50 years and in the United States since the 1970s, thanks to the research done by Dr. John Lee, M.D., and Dr. Jonathon Wright, M.D. There is a multitude of research studies with positive results. Several of these studies are in the resource section at the end of the book.

In the early 1940s, a chemist named Russell Marker discovered a substance found in abundance in the wild yam[1] plant (diosgenin) that could be converted to progesterone and other human hormones. This was a great discovery for women. Marker hoped to ensure a fair price to make it available to all women, so he refused to sign patent rights. Without a patent, pharmaceutical companies are unable to profit from natural hormones. If a drug company is not able to make a potential profit, then they are less willing to put forth the dollars to do research/studies; furthermore, there is no incentive for them to

---

1   Wild yam is different from the sweet potatoes we eat. It is a plant-based estrogen that can be chemically converted into hormones.

help educate women and physicians on the health benefits of bioidentical hormones.

Each bioidentical hormone is compounded to the exact need of an individual because each woman's hormonal system is unique. Compounding pharmacists mix prescriptions to meet each individual's need based upon symptoms and blood and/or saliva testing. Prescriptions can be filled as a cream, gel, pill, sublingual, suppository, or troche (made to dissolve under the tongue). Bioidentical hormones are FDA-approved substances with the same level of guidelines as Premarin® and Provera®. Insurance companies and health plan providers are increasingly covering natural hormone prescriptions, as well as blood testing and saliva testing.

More and more doctors are recommending bioidentical hormones because of their safety and effectiveness. Dr. Uzzi Reiss, M.D., a renowned author and physician in Beverly Hills, believes bioidentical hormones provide an effective and powerful alternative compared to synthetic HRT prescriptions, which consistently cause dangerous side effects in women.

For women to experience optimum health, they need to first find out their current hormone levels. No matter how many or how few hormones need to be adjusted, what I have studied and come to understand, and **resist** is the idea of hormone cocktails, where two or more hormones are filled together as one prescription. Each hormone causes its own symptoms, depending upon whether too little or too much of that hormone is in the body, so hormone cocktails make it difficult to assess which hormone is doing what. Patience and staying in tune with the body's responses are keys to success. When beginning treatment, I recommend taking replacement hormones separately until optimal levels are achieved, and then a cocktail–which could possibly save money–may be considered.

The benefits of natural hormones are so great that it is well worth the effort to find an open-minded, experienced, and caring professional. I have compiled this information to help women understand the how and why of the body's response to hormones, so one can seek out a knowledgeable health professional who can serve as a health care partner. There is no preset formula that will bring good health to everyone. The ways that women eat, exercise, and relax have a major impact on how they feel, so one size does not fit all (or in this case, one prescription).

Research shows that to create proper balance of the endocrine system, first it is necessary to normalize the function of the adrenals and thyroid. The adrenals are part of the major endocrine system. It is imperative for the adrenals to be functioning optimally to maintain healthy homeostasis. As Dr. Eldred Taylor, M.D. says, "We could take estrogen and progesterone all day long and if the adrenals are not working properly, then the entire communication of the endocrine system is broken, and hormone balance is impossible."

Sluggish adrenals over time, slow down the function of the thyroid, thus inhibiting proper stimulation from the thyroid to maintain a proper estrogen/progesterone balance. Proper function of both the adrenals and thyroid are necessary for a balanced hormonal system to be attained.

Toward the end of the book, I go into more detail describing the adrenals and thyroid, their symptoms and treatment, to make sure that your treatment protocol for all your hormones is effective and maintained to achieve overall hormone balance.

CHAPTER 2

PREGNENOLONE

"It's the constant and determined that breaks down all resistance and sweeps away all obstacles."
—Claude M. Bristol

Pregnenolone is the major player in the hierarchy of hormones. It is the first step to hormonal balance. The adrenal gland produces pregnenolone. It is nicknamed the "parent hormone" because it is a precursor to DHEA, which is a precursor to testosterone, estrogen, and progesterone. It is a super-hormone that is the key to keeping the brain functioning at peak capacity, and it falls with age. Pregnenolone is synthesized from cholesterol. The body metabolizes pregnenolone into progesterone and DHEA.

Along with all the other hormones, the pregnenolone level should be tested. It not only enhances the conversion process to other hormones, but it contributes to balancing deficient hormones. Throughout his career, Dr. Reiss has found that optimal pregnenolone levels are not necessarily needed to balance hormones. He states, "I have found that actual blood testing and clinical response does not support the idea that pregnenolone is the source of all hormones. Instead, I have observed that pregnenolone is the key to your brain power." That alone, for me, would be enough reason to take pregnenolone.

Pregnenolone is available as an over-the-counter supplement, but I recommend purchasing it through a compounding pharmacist, where the quality and potency can be trusted. Morning is the suggested time of day for taking pregnenolone because of its energy effect.

BENEFITS OF OPTIMAL LEVELS OF PREGNENOLONE:

- Enhances memory
- Improves concentration
- Has a promising effect on degenerative disorders such as chronic fatigue syndrome, arthritis, lupus, ulcerative colitis, inflammatory bowel disease, Alzheimer's, and connective tissue disorders
- Protects the adrenal glands from stress and mental fatigue
- Helps maintain balance of all hormones (estrogen, progesterone, DHEA, testosterone, etc.)
- Helps relieve arthritic pain
- Enhances the benefit of DHEA
- Helps maintain stamina
- Reduces cholesterol levels
- Increases social confidence
- Helps generate new brain cells
- Repairs nerve regeneration
- Reduces signs of aging skin
- Therapeutic agent for rheumatoid arthritis

Research has shown that pregnenolone even relieves hangovers.

SIGNS OF PREGNENOLONE DEFICIENCIES:

- Dry eyes
- Absent underarm and pubic hair
- Hot flashes
- Fatigue
- Memory loss
- Muscle weakness
- Joint aches and pains

SIGNS OF PREGNENOLONE EXCESS:

- Hyperactivity
- Irritability
- Agitation
- Nervousness

If any of these symptoms occur, reduce the dosage.

Dr. Reiss states that normal levels of pregnenolone in the blood are within the range of 70-120 ng/ml, and the daily recommended dose is 50mg to 100mg. A pill form has a longer lasting effect in the body.

CHAPTER 3

ESTROGEN

estradiol (E2), estrone (E1), estriol (E3)

"He, who has health, has hope.
And he, who has hope, has everything."
—Author unknown

There is no such hormone as estrogen. Estrogen is a class name composed of estradiol (E_2), estrone (E_1), and estriol (E_3). It might be easiest to think of it as a group of hormones that primarily regulate the growth, development, and function of the female reproductive system. Estrogen is produced primarily by the ovaries in addition to fat cells, muscle cells, and skin. It is important to replenish exactly what your body can no longer make. This estrogen combination is compounded in a formula called Tri-Est or Bi-Est. Tri-Est is composed of all three estrogens. Most doctors leave estrone out of the formula because research shows evidence that estrone plays a significant role in breast cancer. The other two major estrogens play a significant role of importance to health and well-being.

Estrogen has a major impact on more than 300 tissue systems throughout the body. Quoting Dr. Reiss, "I am convinced that if a woman maintains a certain level of estrogen, she can delay and somewhat arrest the changes associated with hormonal decline and deficiency." Dr. Lee believes that most women maintain sufficient levels of estrogen even after menopause; therefore, no supplementation is necessary. My observations are that with today's stresses, all of my clients have estrogen levels that are extremely deficient after menopause. This is why testing is so important to determine where your levels are. It allows your physician to help you achieve and maintain hormonal balance.

THE BENEFITS OF ESTROGEN—THE ESSENCE OF FEMININITY:

- Eliminates hot flashes and night sweats
- Maintains hair and skin texture
- Enhances muscle tone
- Reduces wrinkles
- Discomfort from full and tender breasts
- Increases sensuality
- Improves clarity of mind
- Protects against Alzheimer's
- Halts bone loss
- Protects against cardiovascular disease
- Brings a glow to the skin
- Moistens the eyes
- Influences the brain
- Affects vision, hearing, taste, touch, and attention span

ESTRIOL IS THE MOST BENEFICIAL OF THE THREE ESTROGENS:

- Estriol is thought to be protective against breast cancer. As reported by Dr. Alvin Follingstad, "37% of postmenopausal women with metastatic breast cancer who received small doses of estriol had experienced remission or arrest of metastatic tumors."
- Dr. Allen Gaby, M.D., states that estriol protects against thickening of the uterine lining, thus protecting women from postmenopausal vaginal bleeding and endometrial cancer.
- According to Dr. Gaby, "Estriol may also be more effective at lowering the risk of blood clots in the veins or lungs when compared with other estrogens."
- Quoting Dr. Lee: "Estriol is the most active on the vagina, cervix, and vulva. In cases of postmenopausal vaginal dryness and atrophy (tissue breakdown) which predispose a woman to vaginitis and cystitis (bladder infection), estriol supplementation would theoretically be the most effective and safest estrogen to use."
- Dr. Reiss states, "Estriol will enhance vaginal lubrication and elasticity, prevents night sweats, and hot flashes, and promotes the health of the skin."

SIGNS OF ESTROGEN DEFICIENCY:

- Mental fogginess
- Forgetfulness
- Depression
- Minor anxiety (not able to control your worries)
- Mood changes
- Difficulty falling asleep

- Hot flashes
- Night sweats
- Temperature swings
- Day-long fatigue
- Reduced stamina
- Decreased sense of sexuality and sensuality
- Lessened self-image and attention to appearance
- Dry eyes, skin, and vagina
- Loss of skin radiance
- Sense of normalcy only during the second week of the menstrual cycle
- Sagging breasts and loss of fullness
- Pain with sexual activity
- Weight gain, with increasing lack of concern about it
- Increased back and joint pain
- Episodes of rapid heartbeat, with or without anxiety
- Headaches and migraines
- Gastrointestinal discomfort
- Urinary incontinence
- Easily distracted
- Feeling shaky
- Dizziness

The most common symptoms when estrogen levels fall are hot flashes, inability to sleep, mental fogginess, and emotional instability. Surprisingly, as soon as replacement begins, you can see a difference within 30 minutes to 1-1/2 hours after giving the body what it has been missing: **ESTROGEN.**

COMMON SIGNS OF ESTROGEN DOMINANCE:

- Breast tenderness or pain
- Increased breast size

- Water retention
- Impatient, snappy behavior, but with a clear mind
- Pelvic cramps, with or without uterine bleeding
- Nausea
- PMS
- Mood swings
- Anxiety
- Irritability
- Headaches
- Heavy or irregular bleeding
- Weight gain in hips and fat storage
- Bloating
- Changes in libido
- Craving sweets
- Depression
- Growth of uterine lining
- Growth of breast tissue
- Thickening of the blood (hypercoagulability)
- Thyroid dysfunction

DANGERS OF ESTROGEN DOMINANCE:

- Greater incidence of breast, ovarian, and uterine cancer
- Endometriosis
- Uterine fibroids and polyps
- Adenomyosis (benign growths of the lining of the uterus into the muscle wall, which is very painful)
- Fibrocystic breast disease
- Thickening of the uterus which can lead to endometrial cancer

WAYS TO APPLY ESTROGEN:

- **Transdermal Bi-Est Cream (combination of estradiol and estriol):** Where to apply estrogen cream is a controversy. Some physicians, like Dr. Lee, believe that Bi-Est should be applied to thin areas such as palms, inner arms, and backs of knees. Other doctors believe that the cream should be applied to thicker skin areas such as buttocks, inner thighs, and low stomach. I suggest discussing this with your doctor to find the most effective method. Avoid putting estrogen on the breast, neck, and face. Saliva testing is more accurate with this method.
- **Sublingual:** Place drops or lozenges under the tongue and allow to dissolve. This way of delivery enters the body quickly but also leaves the body quickly. Serum testing is most accurate with this method.
- **Patches of Estradiol:** Commercially made patches placed on the skin transmit a continuous release of estradiol. When used with progesterone, patches do not present a high risk of cancer, but the body is losing out on the wonderful benefits of estriol that can be compounded in the prescription Bi-Est. On a personal note, stay tuned in to your body when using patches because side effects can occur such as weight gain, backache, headache, or a skin rash. Always remember: Never use estrogen without progesterone.
- **Oral (pill form):** Research shows that oral estrogen increases C-reactive protein (CRP), a marker of inflammation that is associated with heart disease. It has also been associated with dementia and urinary incontinence. I suggest never using estrogen orally until other forms of delivery have been tried. If the body does not absorb estrogen using the other forms of delivery, then it may be necessary to take it orally.

CHAPTER 4

PROGESTERONE

(The Counterpart of Estrogen)

"There is nothing mysterious about aging.
Aging is simply an inherited hormonal
neuroendocrine program ... that can be
modified, delayed, or reversed."
—Walter Pierpaoli, M.D.

It is critical to keep progesterone and estrogen in balance. Progesterone should be considered a lifelong partner of estrogen. Progesterone is a precursor hormone, meaning it is essential to enhance other hormones such as estrogen and testosterone. Progesterone levels need to be at optimum levels throughout a woman's lifetime.

During pregnancy, women have an abundance of progesterone, and for the most part, feel their best. As women age, progesterone levels drastically fall. In fact, by the age of 35, most women are deficient; therefore, estrogen is dominant. Menopausal women are usually extremely progesterone deficient. Dr. Jesse Lynn Hanley, states, "It may be the single most powerful agent at a woman's disposal that is also simple, appropriate, and doesn't require lifestyle changes."

I have been coaching several young women in their twenties, and their test results are showing that, even at this young age, they are already estrogen dominant. I believe that young women should have all their hormones tested, especially progesterone. This way, they can treat estrogen dominance or any other imbalance, early. We need to promote wellness by teaching prevention and self-care. Getting to the root cause of disease helps patients maintain optimal wellness, and treating hormonal imbalance at a very young age could prevent disease and save lives. Again, I want to emphasize: It is extremely important never to use estrogen without progesterone. Balance is the key!

BENEFITS OF PROGESTERONE:

- Promotes the buildup of new bone tissue
- Produces a calming, mild tranquilizing effect
- Enhances an overall sense of well-being
- Protects the breast, uterus, and probably the ovaries from cancer
- Acts as a natural diuretic
- Decreases PMS and menstrual flow
- Enhances the body's defenses
- Improves the breakdown of fat into energy
- Cuts the craving for carbohydrates and sweets
- Reduces breast tenderness and pain
- Increases HDL, the body's "good cholesterol"
- Reduces anxiety
- Decreases estrogen receptors that cause breast cancer
- Balances estrogen

- Re-grows scalp hair
- Protects against thickening of the uterus which can lead to endometrial cancer

COMMON SIGNS OF PROGESTERONE DEFICIENCY:

- Anxiety, irritability, and nervousness
- Water retention
- Amenorrhea—absence of ovulation and menstruation; the ovaries are producing only a bare minimum of progesterone
- Oligomenorrhea—infrequent periods, perhaps every few months
- Heavy and frequent periods—related to tissue buildup in the uterus because of prolonged progesterone deficiency
- Spotting a few days before the periods—progesterone level is dropping rapidly and prematurely during the monthly cycle
- PMS—most symptoms of premenstrual syndrome, whether physical or emotional, relate to the lack of progesterone
- Cystic breasts, breasts with lumps
- Painful breasts
- Endometriosis and adenomyosis (a benign inward growth of the lining of the uterus into the muscle wall that is very painful)
- Fibroids
- Headaches, migraines
- Feeling withdrawn
- Pelvic pain
- Fainting spells
- Abdominal bloating
- Acne below the mouth, on the cheeks, and temples

- Frequent urination
- Craving specific foods, especially chocolate or sweets
- Lack of libido
- Mental confusion
- Feeling aggressive
- Feeling shaky
- Insomnia
- Lethargy
- Depression
- Crying for no apparent reason
- Night sweats just before your period
- Urinary incontinence

As you probably have observed, deficient progesterone symptoms are very similar to dominant estrogen symptoms.

DANGERS OF PROGESTERONE DEFICIENCY:

- Uterine cancer
- Thickening of the uterus, which can lead to endometrial cancer
- Osteoporosis
- Heart disease and depression
- Polycystic ovary syndrome (PCOS)
- Cysts on the ovaries

SIGNS OF EXCESS PROGESTERONE:

Mild Reactions:

- Drowsiness
- Slight dizziness

- Increased agitation
- Water retention
- Very few women may experience a toxic response
- Nausea
- Fatigue

If any of these symptoms occur, simply decrease your dosage.

WAYS TO TAKE PROGESTERONE:

- **Prometrium Capsules** are made of peanut oil. There is good news and not-so-good news for this method of delivery. It is great for calming, and it helps to promote a good night's sleep, but it will go through the liver before being used by the body, and only 40% or less of the dosage may be absorbed.
- **Sublingual Drops or Troches** (lozenges) are placed under the tongue. This method enters the body immediately but also leaves the body quickly. If serum levels are being used, they are more accurate with this method.
- **Topical Cream**—Dr. Lee says to apply it everywhere you blush: your face, palms of your hands, back of your hands, chest, inner thighs, outer thighs, back of knees, and breasts. He says the places on your body where you blush are where you have the most capillaries. Therefore, absorption is better because the capillaries are the closest to the surface. Always rotate application each time for best absorption and to reach a stable level. Research shows that this is the most effective form of delivery. Progesterone cream should be applied two times a day for best results. Saliva testing shows more accurate levels for this method.

- **Over-The-Counter Creams** are of a low concentration and usually not strong enough to bring progesterone to optimal levels. If they work, the deficiency is minimal.

Whatever form of delivery is used, always monitor your intake with a physician.

CHAPTER 5

TESTOSTERONE

"Life should not be defined by age, but by energy. Aging equates to disease. Energy equates to health."
—Michael Galitzer, M.D.

Testosterone is an androgen hormone (a male sex hormone) produced in both men and women. Levels peak around the age of 25 and then slowly decline. Although women produce less testosterone than men, it still plays a very important role in their health. Studies have shown that women who use testosterone report a renewed sense of vitality, increased libido, and improvement in overall sense of well-being. Testosterone needs to be balanced in both men and women. It needs to stay at appropriate levels to protect against prostate cancer. Research shows that if men brought their levels of testosterone to optimal levels at the first sign of deficiency, they could head off prostate cancer.

BENEFITS OF OPTIMAL LEVELS OF TESTOSTERONE:

- Increases bone density and bone formation

- Enhances energy, sex drive, orgasmic power, and enhanced emotional aspect of sexuality
- Decreases body fat
- Increases bone and muscle strength
- Lowers blood pressure
- Modulates levels of LDL and HDL
- Keeps a woman's skin soft and supple
- Protects against plaque in the blood vessels
- Improves balance and hand-to-eye coordination
- Helps the body recover from physical stress
- Alleviates "cluster" headaches when combined with melatonin and estrogen
- Enhances the feeling of well-being and self-esteem

SIGNS OF TESTOSTERONE DEFICIENCIES:

- Flabbiness and muscular weakness, as in sagging upper arms and cheeks
- Loss of hair on the head
- Lack of energy and stamina
- Loss of coordination and balance
- Loss of sense of security
- Indecisiveness
- Decreased sex drive
- Poor body image
- Decreased armpit, pubic, and body hair
- Urinary incontinence
- Facial hair

SIGNS OF TESTOSTERONE EXCESS:

- Hostility
- Angry outbursts
- Feeling aggressive
- Lack of libido
- Muscle pain
- Weight gain
- Wasting away (or loss) of muscle tone and mass
- Acne
- Excess facial and body hair
- Depression
- Irritability

SUPPLEMENTING TESTOSTERONE:

- **Gel or Cream Form**—These are suggested to be the best forms of delivery:
  1. Apply either to the right or left inner thigh. This benefits the whole body, including the bones, muscles, cardiovascular system, and emotional health.
  2. Apply to the hairless area between the vagina and the rectum. This serves and restores the bladder muscle, the sexual organs, and the pelvic muscles.
  3. Apply to the labia. This targets the vagina more precisely.
- **Sublingual Drops or Troche (under the tongue):** As noted previously, blood testing is more accurate with this method.

Dosage differs from one individual to the next and depends on what you and your doctor agrees is the best treatment for you.

CHAPTER 6

DHEA

(DEHYDROEPIANDROSTERONE)

*"Knowing you are at risk empowers you to
do things that can greatly lessen the chance
of developing diabetes or heart disease."*
—Geoffrey Redmond, M.D.

DHEA is the most abundant hormone in the body. It is referred to as "the feel-good hormone" and is nicknamed the "Mother of all Hormones" because of its ability to convert into estrogen and testosterone. It is produced by the adrenal glands, the glands that make adrenaline and cortisol. It reaches its peak in the teen years. As we age, DHEA declines rapidly. Clinical studies have proven that DHEA has a profound effect on the immune system, sex drive, metabolism, and one's own emotional stability. Dr. Neil Rouzier M.D. states, "DHEA is definitely one hormone we should never let slip to low levels. It has been shown to inhibit disease, preserve youth, and maintain health." Baseline blood testing of DHEAS should be done prior to starting on DHEA. Forms of delivery include capsule, sublingual, or transdermal cream. Regular monitoring of blood levels is recommended, as with all hormones.

BENEFITS OF OPTIMAL LEVELS OF DHEA:

- Improves energy and stamina
- Protects against breast cancer
- Enhances the immune system
- Enhances metabolism
- Helps the body cope with stress and anxiety
- Maintains a healthy sex drive
- Decreases depression
- Alters cognitive decline
- Maintains mental alertness
- Protects against diabetes
- Exerts a healthy influence over the heart, lowering cholesterol, and preventing blood clots
- Optimal levels of DHEA in the body have been associated with lower incidence of cancer
- Improves skin wound healing
- Reduces osteoarthritis and joint pain
- Maintains collagen levels in the skin, promoting smoother, younger-looking skin
- Reduces free radicals in the body
- Enhances a feeling of well-being
- Improves bone strength
- Stabilizes blood sugar levels
- Protects against the development of the metabolic insulin resistance syndrome
- Reduces abdominal fat
- Increases muscle mass and strength

The scientific community and the Mayo Clinic are undertaking research of DHEA for its proposed benefits for several medical conditions such as systemic depression, connective tissue disease, adrenal insufficiency, and more. With all the research I have done, I feel confident that there is promise that the FDA will approve DHEA for these medical conditions.

SIGNS OF DHEA DEFICIENCY:

- Anxiety
- Lack of stamina
- Intolerance to loud noise
- Constant fatigue
- Mood swings
- Compromised immune system
- Memory loss
- Lack of pubic hair
- Poor abdominal muscle support
- Dry skin and eyes
- Poor sex drive
- Depression
- Mental confusion
- Joint pain and swelling
- Lack of focus, easily distracted

SIGNS OF DHEA EXCESS:

- Oily skin
- Increased facial and body hair
- Polycystic ovary syndrome (a hormonal defect that causes an over-production of DHEA and testosterone), usually caused in childbirth
- Becoming edgy and irritable

DHEA DEFICIENCY IS FOUND IN ALMOST EVERY MAJOR CATEGORY OF DISEASE:

- Lupus
- Rheumatoid Arthritis
- Multiple Sclerosis
- Chronic Fatigue Syndrome
- AIDS
- Allergies
- Osteoporosis
- Alzheimer's disease
- Obesity
- High blood pressure
- Heart disease
- Diabetes
- Thyroid disease

CHAPTER 7

MELATONIN

*"A wise man ought to realize that health
is his most valuable possession."*
—Author unknown

Melatonin is a natural hormone produced in the pineal gland which is in the deepest part of the human brain. It regulates the circadian rhythm (the sleep, wake cycle) and also correlates with a number of other functions and problems in the body. As we age, we produce less melatonin. There is research showing that melatonin is one of the safest and least toxic hormones to take, and is often suggested for anyone over the age of 40. Melatonin may extend our life span more than 25%, which may be because it is a very powerful antioxidant. Dr. Reiss suggests that those with autoimmune disorders or a compromised immune system or adrenal insufficiency should be cautious taking melatonin because it affects the production of other hormones. If you are extremely stressed and fatigued, you should discuss tests that should be done to determine adrenal insufficiency. If you do not have adrenal fatigue or an autoimmune disease, then research shows, if tolerated, even large doses of melatonin are harmless.

BENEFITS OF MELATONIN:

- Promotes healthy sleep
- Relieves jet lag by resetting the body clock
- Used as a preventive for cancers, most notably colon, ovarian, prostate, melanoma, and most recently, breast cancer
- Lowers cholesterol
- Is a powerful antioxidant
- Promotes zinc utilization
- Promotes the production of T3
- Enhances sexual function
- Slows down the aging process
- Improves immune system
- Improves mood
- Promotes cardiovascular health by reducing the "bad" LDL cholesterol
- Used as a treatment for prostate enlargement
- Helps treat tinnitus
- Decreases migraines
- Protects the liver and kidneys through its anti-inflammatory effect
- Improves and resolves dry eye syndrome
- Protects DNA
- Reduces blood coagulation
- Positive influence on our hormones and nervous system

DANGERS OF HIGH DOSES OF MELATONIN:

- Insomnia (this also happens if adrenal fatigue is present)
- Nightmares rather than peaceful sleep
- Headaches
- Mental impairment

- Dizziness
- Day time sleepiness
- Crankiness
- Drugs that suppress the immune system

DRUGS THAT MELATONIN MAY BE CONTRAINDICATED:

- Blood-thinning medications
- Drugs that suppress the immune system
- Diabetes drugs
- Birth control pills

I suggest you do your own research and I highly encourage you to work with a knowledgeable healthcare practitioner when taking melatonin or any other hormone, even if it is available over the counter at health food stores.

CHAPTER 8

THYROID HORMONE

"If someone does not feel well or, to be more direct, cannot enjoy life she is entitled to help— even if her condition is not defined in a textbook and even if her lab results are normal."
—Geoffrey Redmond, M.D.

The thyroid is a small butterfly-shaped gland located in the front of the neck. It is a very complex organ that is a major player in hormonal function. The thyroid gland is the body's metabolic thermostat. It influences essentially every organ, tissue, and cell in the body. According to the American Thyroid Association, 27 million Americans have an overactive (hyperthyroid) or underactive (hypothyroid) gland.

It is very important to make sure your thyroid is functioning optimally before beginning any hormonal replacement program. To get the most accurate picture of how your thyroid is performing, the basic blood tests you can ask your doctor to do are thyroid stimulating hormone (TSH), triiodothyronine (T3 Free), thyroxine (T4 free), and triiodothyronine T3 reverse (rT3). The thyroid peroxidase antibody (TPO) is also recommended to diagnose the possibility of Hashimoto's thyroiditis, a thyroid autoimmune disease.

If blood tests come back normal, encourage your doctor to look further, and to please listen to all your symptoms. Medical history, family history, physical examination, and measurement of the basal temperature of the body must be considered to obtain a proper diagnosis. If you have many symptoms of hypothyroidism and your tests come back normal, but your doctor will not treat you, then look for another doctor who will listen. If they fail to do the necessary testing, then see a functional medicine doctor. They will look at you as a whole person and definitely treat your thyroid properly. Your health depends on your thyroid working at optimal levels. Note: If your thyroid fails, so, in turn, will you.

COMMON SYMPTOMS OF HYPOTHYROIDISM:

- Fatigue
- Forgetfulness
- Depression
- Heavy menses
- Dry, coarse hair
- Mood swings
- Weight gain
- Hoarseness
- Dry, coarse skin
- Constipation
- Ridges on your nails
- Brittle nails
- Cold intolerance
- Difficulty swallowing
- Eyelid swelling
- Hair loss
- Muscle weakness
- Puffy eyes

- Nervousness
- Loss of hair on outer third of eyebrows
- Irritability
- Menstrual irregularities
- Bloating

COMMON SYMPTOMS OF HYPERTHYROIDISM:

- Heat intolerance, sweating
- Weight loss
- Change in appetite
- Frequent bowel movements
- Changes in vision
- Fatigue and muscle weakness
- Menstrual disturbances
- Mental disturbances
- Sleep disturbances
- Tremors
- Thyroid enlargement (goiter)

RESULTS IF THYROID GOES UNTREATED:

- High serum cholesterol
- Atherosclerosis
- Osteoporosis
- Circulatory and cardiovascular disease
- Infertility

TWO TREATMENTS FOR THYROID DISEASE:

Synthroid® is the drug of choice by most conventional physicians. Although there is a lot of research to back up their choice, it is a synthetic drug that only contains T4. The thyroid gland is made up of two hormones: T3 and T4.

Armour®, Nature-throid®, and WP Thyroid® are all desiccated thyroid hormone brands and found to be the most effective thyroid hormone replacement. Desiccated thyroid requires a prescription and is regulated by the FDA. It has been used for more than 100 years. It is derived from the thyroid gland of the pig and is the closest comparative to the human thyroid gland. It contains both thyroid hormones, T4 and T3. T3 is the active hormone. I refer to T3 as the energy part of the hormone. T4 must convert to T3. When one's immune system is compromised, the body can lose the ability to make this conversion, which is the most important process necessary to regulate thyroid function.

Proper replacement is imperative for optimal thyroid function. Each brand varies in price, and one may be more effective for you than another. Work with your practitioner to figure out which is best for you. You may find it very helpful to research Dr. Wilson's Syndrome, concerning the treatment of the thyroid with T3. His website can be found in the resource section in the back of this book.

This is some very basic information on the thyroid gland. I urge you to do your own research if you have any of the symptoms listed above. There is so much more to know about the function of your thyroid gland.

CHAPTER 9

IODINE AND THYROID FUNCTION

"Half the costs of illness are wasted on conditions that could be prevented."
—Dr. Joseph Pizzorno

Iodine is the essential chemical needed for your thyroid to work optimally. Dr. David Brownstein, M.D., has dedicated many years researching the importance of iodine in the body. Iodine is found in each of the trillions of cells in the body. If we do not have adequate levels of iodine in our system, then life itself is not possible.

Your body needs iodine to make the thyroid hormone. A deficient level of iodine in the body may cause a sluggish thyroid and possibly a goiter (an enlarged thyroid). The thyroid hormone must be able to convert from the inactive part of the thyroid (T4) to the active part of the thyroid (T3) for you to have optimal thyroid function. Iodine allows the conversion to take place. Unfortunately, there is not a really good test for iodine, so my personal recommendation is to see an alternative doctor like one of the two kinesiologists that I mention in the resource section in the back of this book.

Dr. Brownstein states, "It is almost impossible to have a balanced endocrine system without having adequate iodine in your system." Iodine is not just necessary for proper thyroid function; it is also responsible for the production of all the other hormones of the body. The main source of iodine comes from ocean foods and salt. For many reasons, iodine is not adequate in our food supply. Iodine deficiency has a definite connection to breast cancer. Research is showing that an iodine epidemic is coming to the forefront as in the 1960s. Correcting iodine deficiency has proven to have many positive health benefits.

IODINE DEFICIENCY DISORDERS:

- Goiter (enlarged thyroid)
- Mental retardation
- Infertility
- Increased child and infant mortality

ADEQUATE LEVELS OF IODINE ARE NECESSARY FOR:

- Proper immune system function
- Protection against antibacterial or parasitic infection
- Protection against viruses
- Protection against many cancers
- Adequate conversion of T4 into T3
- Optimal functioning of all glands

CONDITIONS TREATED WITH IODINE:

- ADD
- Breast disease
- Excess mucous production
- Fatigue
- Fibrocystic breasts
- Hemorrhoids
- Headaches
- Keloids
- Ovarian disease
- Thyroid disorders
- Vaginal infections
- Sebaceous cysts
- Autoimmune illnesses
- Thyroid conditions
- Fibrocystic breasts
- Ovarian cysts
- Hair loss

CHAPTER 10

HEALTHY ADRENAL GLANDS

"Ignoring your body—thinking it will just somehow take care of itself or putting your health care completely in the hands of others—can have serious consequences."
—Uzzi Reiss, M.D., O.B./GYN

The adrenals are two small glands that sit on top of the kidneys. They play a significant part in regulating many bodily functions, specifically hormonal function. One critical hormone that is produced by the adrenal glands is cortisol. According to Dr. Williams McK Jefferies M.D., **"CORTISOL IS THE ONLY HORMONE THAT IS ABSOLUTELY ESSENTIAL FOR LIFE."** Chronic prolonged stress forces the adrenals to release continuous cortisol, which leads to adrenal insufficiency, causing hormonal imbalances. Unfortunately, Western medicine only treats disease, so unless you have Addison's disease (hypoadrenia) or Cushing's disease (extremely high levels of cortisol caused mostly by steroid drugs), there is very little attention given to the patient with symptoms of adrenal insufficiency. Because endocrinologists rarely recognize adrenal fatigue as a distinct condition, they are, in turn, unprepared to treat it as one. All dynamic functions in the body need cortisol.

ADRENAL GLAND FUNCTION:

- Affects stability in energy levels
- Maintains physical and emotional stamina
- Affects stability of body temperature
- Supports heart and blood pressure
- Helps prevent PMS
- Affects integrity of bone density, joints, and muscles
- Affects the stability of glucose regulation and digestive processes
- Supports the immune and nervous system
- Helps prevent depression and maintains emotional stability
- Helps maintain skin integrity and texture
- Affects stability of optimal body weight
- Helps prevent miscarriages
- Helps prevent dysmenorrheal (absent) or painful periods

SYMPTOMS OF ADRENAL INSUFFICIENCY OR ADRENAL EXHAUSTION:

- Unstable blood sugar
- Mood swings
- Foggy thinking
- Hormone resistance, especially DHEA and progesterone
- Acne, worse with menses
- Alcohol intolerance

- Allergies
- Chronic illness
- Depression
- Fatigue
- Dry, thin skin
- Hair loss
- Low blood pressure
- Hypoglycemia
- Lightheadedness
- Low body temperature
- Dizziness when standing
- Thyroid dysfunction

If you feel run down and basically lousy, and have several of the symptoms noted above, share these symptoms with your doctor. You will probably need to find a holistic doctor, functional medicine doctor, endocrinologist, or your family medical doctor who recognizes adrenal insufficiency and treats with an integrative approach. Trust me that it will be well worth your time. When your adrenals are well, your whole body functions optimally. I highly suggest you read *Adrenal Fatigue, The 21st Century Stress Syndrome* by James L. Wilson, N.D., D.C., Ph.D. Dr. Wilson has done a lot of research on the treatment of adrenal disorders and has his own protocol for stabilizing adrenal function.

FOLLOWING ARE SOME DIETARY SUPPLEMENTS THAT PLAY AN IMPORTANT ROLE IN HEALING ADRENAL FATIGUE:

- Vitamin C
- Vitamin E
- B Complex vitamins

- Magnesium
- Calcium
- Trace minerals
- B6 and B12
- Folate
- Zinc
- Selenium

Working with a qualified health care practitioner to assure proper dosing of supplements is greatly advised.

There are medical tests available to help diagnose adrenal insufficiency but, remember, these tests diagnose disease (Addison's or Cushing's disease). I have always said you have to be nearly dead before tests show a problem and unfortunately, this is truer than you realize. Ask your doctor to perform:

- ACTH serum test (Adrenocorticotropic Hormone)
- A new sensitive ACTH (Cortrosyn Stimulation Test)
- 24-hour urine test
- Morning cortisol

Along with medical tests, research shows the very best indicator of adrenal insufficiency is a saliva test. You can obtain this test from your gynecologist, endocrinologist, or compounding pharmacist. At the end of this book, I reference where to get a saliva test online. Borrow from the library a book by Dr. Jefferies M.D., *Safe Uses of Cortisol*. Dr. Jefferies has dedicated many years researching the benefits of hydrocortisone using physiological doses. This book is full of information and research studies. It became my Bible for referencing my adrenal problems as well as my daughter's. The information I received from this book changed my life.

Another great resource for adrenal help is Dr. Lam's book, *Adrenal Fatigue Syndrome*. It is the latest and most up-to-date information and research on all stages of adrenal fatigue. He is an expert in the field and works with patients on a personal basis. Check out his website. The resource section in the back of this book contains the reference.

CHAPTER 11

VITAMIN D

"We age because our hormones decline; our hormones don't decline because we age."
—Suzanne Somers

Lately, a lot of attention is being given to the necessity of optimal levels of Vitamin D. Due to its structure and mechanism of action, it resembles more of a hormone than that of a vitamin. It occurs in nature in two main forms: Vitamin D2 and D3. Both are converted into 25-hydroxyvitamin D, the primary circulating form of Vitamin D. Most of us do not get enough vitamin D through sun exposure or foods; therefore, supplementation is necessary. Vitamin D's most crucial role is regulating calcium and phosphorus concentrations in the serum. The Institute of Medicine established the upper limit of Vitamin D to be 2,000 IU per day.

I am finding that most of my clients need 5,000 IU per day to get their lab values above 50. Personally, with all the research I have done, I am finding that supplementation of Vitamin D warrants more IU for optimal health, so I take 5,000 IU/daily and keep my lab values close to 70. Recent trials in healthy adults have found no evidence of toxicity at doses less than 10,000 IU/daily and lab values less than 100.

Excessive Vitamin D intake could result in increased blood calcium levels. The effects of this may be gastrointestinal symptoms, depression, confusion, kidney stones, and more frequent urination.

We are looking at an epidemic of Vitamin D deficiency in the U.S., so it is crucial for you to ask your doctor to check your Vitamin D level regularly. The test to ask for is a 25-Hydroxyvitamin D3 serum. Very low levels of Vitamin D are being treated with injections. The best form of Vitamin D to take is D3. Please get yours checked today!

VITAMIN D PLAYS A MAJOR ROLE IN PREVENTING THESE CANCERS:

- Colon
- Breast
- Prostate
- Ovarian
- Esophageal
- Renal
- Bladder
- Lung
- Pancreatic

OTHER DISEASES AND HEALTH CONCERNS WHERE VITAMIN D PLAYS MAJOR ROLE IN PREVENTION AND HEALING:

- Osteoporosis
- Autoimmune disease (multiple sclerosis)
- Type 1 diabetes

- Insulin resistance
- Leg weakness
- Muscle wasting
- Dental health
- Musculoskeletal pain
- Stroke
- Hypertension
- Skin disorders (psoriasis)
- Metabolic syndrome
- Influenza

CHAPTER 12

TESTS TO DO BEFORE BEGINNING BIOIDENTICAL HORMONES

If women don't educate themselves – and, if necessary, educate their doctors – they can be subject to spectacular mistreatment."
—Marcus Laux, N.D.

BEFORE YOU BEGIN TAKING HORMONES, WHETHER IT IS ONE OR MULTIPLE, DISCUSS THESE TESTS AND EXAMS WITH YOUR DOCTOR:

- Have a physical and gynecological check-up including breast exam, mammogram, or thermogram, and pap smear. If your breasts are dense, ask about a thermogram, digital testing, ultrasound, or MRI. Please do not just keep getting mammograms if you have dense breasts.

Discuss with your doctor what diagnostic test may be more appropriate for you.

- Women in early menopause should check their Follicle Stimulating Hormone (FSH) level to confirm the diagnosis of menopause.
- Full cardiovascular testing should be done prior to hormonal treatment, including a high sensitivity C-reactive protein (hs-CRP) and homocysteine levels. A (hs-CRP) is a protein found in the blood which signals inflammation of the arteries, a potential precursor of a heart attack. High levels of the amino acid homocysteine are linked to heart disease.
- A pelvic transvaginal ultrasound is needed to get a baseline for the thickness of the uterine lining. This helps identify a problem if one should arise. If we know the thickness of the lining before hormonal treatment, then we can easily identify if estrogen replacement is cited as the cause of something suspicious, or if there was a pre-existing condition. A woman's endometrial lining that is higher than 5 millimeters is suspicious, and further evaluation is needed. This is also an opportune time to rule out any polyps or fibroids. Monitoring your uterine lining every two years with an ultrasound is highly recommended.
- Have all hormonal blood levels drawn, or do complete saliva testing of hormones, including morning cortisol and thyroid levels. These tests should be used as guidelines. Find a doctor who will listen closely to your symptoms and treat you appropriately.
- Dr. Reiss encourages women to get a baseline level of SHBG (sex hormone binding globulin). SHBG is a protective protein produced by the liver when it is affected by estrogen. When estrogen is too high, your liver pumps out extra SHBG. This special protein binds

up estrogen and testosterone, resulting in a deficiency in these important hormones. Stress can also cause your SHBG to go up, causing a deficiency in important hormones, and not allowing for optimal benefits. I urge you to make this a part of your hormonal work-up. Compounding gels or creams bind up less estrogen than sublingual application. SHBG may be the key to achieving overall hormonal balance. A blood test can monitor levels of SHBG in your body. The blood level should be no higher than 100. If it is over 100 and you're using capsules or sublinguals for estrogen and/ or testosterone, switch to a gel or cream. If it is over 100 and you are using a gel or cream, use less.

TO HELP SIMPLIFY THINGS FOR YOU, HERE IS A LIST OF TESTS THAT MANY DOCTORS BELIEVE SHOULD BE DONE BEFORE YOU START ON A HORMONAL PROGRAM. IT IS IMPORTANT TO GET A BASELINE OF ALL YOUR HORMONES:

- Progesterone
- Pregnenolone
- Estradiol
- Estriol
- Estrone
- Testosterone – total and free
- DHEA-S
- Sex hormone binding globulin (SHBG)
- TSH
- T3 Free
- T4 Free
- Serum reverse T3
- Thyroid peroxidase antibody (TPO)

- 25 Hydroxy D3
- B12
- Cortisol
- High-sensitive C-reactive protein (CRP)
- Homocysteine plasma
- Lipid panel
- CBC
- Metabolic panel
- FSH and LH (if not menopausal)

CHAPTER 13

TESTIMONIALS

*"I believe that prevention
is the ultimate key to longevity."*
—Neal Rouzier, M.D.

Here are testimonials of a few women who I have coached so they could reap the wonderful benefits of bioidentical hormones.

LYN:

Since I have been into alternative medical therapies for many years (even for my dogs) and I read a lot, I knew my choice would not be synthetic hormones when going through my menopausal transition. I had also been diagnosed with osteoporosis at age 50, and, against my better judgment, was taking Actonel®. A DEXA scan one year later showed severe osteoporosis! I began researching alternative therapies for this and found Susan on a website for osteoporosis, and I thank heaven I did.

My ob/gyn physician of a few years didn't believe in bioidentical hormones, and I was feeling very frustrated researching doctors in New Jersey who specialized in this field. With Susan's help and my newfound hormone knowledge, I was empowered to go to my former ob/gyn physician who is now working with me. If I didn't have Susan to educate me on the benefits of bioidentical hormones, what blood work to do, make suggestions as to where my hormone levels should be, etc., I would never be in the "balanced" state that I am in today. Susan even spoke to my compounding pharmacist to go over my blood work results.

It has only been a couple of months, but I am able to sleep soundly and have an overall feeling of calmness and many other benefits (wink, wink). I also know that these hormones are stopping my bone loss and rebuilding bone. Susan is a lifesaver and my hormone "guru." Even though I live far away, I know I can always count on her to help with any questions I may have (which are many). She checks on me regularly and is such a pleasure and joy to work with, and has a wealth of knowledge when it comes to getting women back to their balanced hormonal state. So grateful!

GAIL:

I would never want to be without our current advances in medicine, but it is also important to understand other approaches that help a person to achieve health and wellness.

Thanks to Susan, I have become more cognizant of natural approaches to anti-aging.

Early in 2011, I felt lower both emotionally and physically than I had at any point in my life. To my dismay, all the doctors prescribed were anti-depressants and sleeping pills.

As a practicing psychologist, I knew my mood might have been low, but I knew depression was not the cause of my problems; it was only a SYMPTOM of something underlying.

I am grateful to have found Susan Berkey. We began to work with a supportive and caring M.D. With Susan's recommendations for blood work and vitamin regimen, I felt for the first time I was in good hands. My blood work found low levels of progesterone and vitamin D, both were addressed, and now my levels are great. At 51 years old, I take no pharmaceuticals, feel, and look great. Bioidentical hormones, supplements, exercise, a good diet, and anti-aging research are my first line of defense to personal health and wellness.

Thank you, Susan, for giving me the knowledge and guidance so I can continue my quest for good health.

BRENDA:

At age 42, I started menopause. At first, I thought it was stress from work and our hectic family life. I thought 42 was too "young" to start menopause, and then my cycle just stopped. I was so involved with my family and job that I never really spent the time studying hormones like I should have, like we all should. I began to drag and just didn't feel well anymore. I went back and forth with my doctor regarding hormone replacement therapy. He kept touting the need for HRT (heart, bones, memory), and I finally gave in for a short period of time trying Premarin®. Instead of feeling better, I had more symptoms: bloating, water retention, mood swings, etc.

Susan has always been focused on health-related issues and would direct articles to me to read. She has made bioidentical hormone research her mantra. Susan is extremely knowledgeable regarding the function of all the hormones and their recommended levels. We finally found a doctor knowledgeable about bioidentical hormones, so, she gladly went with me to my first appointment to assist in helping make accurate replacement values based upon my serum levels. I am extremely grateful for Susan's support because I don't know how many more years it would have taken me to make the move. I was already 55 when I started bioidentical hormones.

I feel so much better now. For the first time in many, many years, I get a great night's sleep and actually dream again. I am anxious to see how much improvement there will be when I have my next bone density test. My only regret is that I didn't make the move 13 years ago! I was lucky enough to have Susan accompany me to my doctor's visit, but since this is not practical for everyone, Susan's summation of her research will be a great tool for every woman to take with her to their doctor to discuss the wonderful benefits of bioidentical hormone therapy. Thank you, Susan!

CHERYL:

I have Susan to thank for convincing me to address my symptoms of hormonal imbalance. To her credit, she has done all the research. She is an expert on the subject of hormone balance and the synergistic effects on how one hormone affects another. The women's health study scared me, and I immediately ceased using the synthetic hormones that the ob/gyn, of course, had prescribed. I began my journey through menopause at that point of "Cold Turkey." Of course, I was using the over-the-counter supplements and soy milk in an effort to combat the hot flashes, insomnia, weight gain, lethargy, and to regain some type of sex life. Armed with what I read in Suzanne Somers' book and my numerous discussions with Susan, I decided to take further action. Susan enlightened me to the idea of bioidentical hormone replacement therapy. In 2004, I sought out the services of a local holistic M.D. whose entire practice is devoted to helping women and men through the hormonal imbalance crisis. Within weeks of taking specific compounded bioidentical hormones, all my hormonal symptoms subsided. Today, I have energy to burn. I sleep throughout the night. Night sweats are a distant memory, and my sex life has returned. Thank you, Susan and Suzanne, you saved my life!

MARTA:

In early menopause, I was concerned about my bone loss, stress-related symptoms, and other menopausal symptoms. My ob/gyn offered no natural treatment plan. My dear friend, Susan, has researched bioidentical hormones for many, many years, so I consulted her. Susan introduced me to a doctor who is knowledgeable in the field of natural hormones. She gave me the knowledge that I needed to feel comfortable talking to my ob/gyn as a partnership and as a team, and I was able to get the help I needed. Susan suggested blood work as well as saliva testing that would be beneficial. She even accompanied me to my doctor appointments. Together, we reviewed the results and developed a treatment plan. Today I feel great! I am excited that my bones have remained stable. I believe I have progesterone to thank for that. I definitely feel less stressed, and I have a lot more energy. I feel confident that I will feel great for many years to come, thanks to Susan's knowledge and assistance.

CHAPTER 14

HORMONES AND DIET

*"It is up to you to be an informed patient.
You must know your stuff and you must have
questions ready that you want answered when
you are with your doctor. We are living in a new
and changed world; we are on our own."*
—Suzanne Somers

This last section is devoted to the importance of diet.
Consuming fruits and vegetables is essential to receiving the
proper antioxidants. You can take bioidentical hormones and
get plenty of exercise, but without a proper diet, you will
likely fail to obtain your health goals. A good diet full of fruits
and vegetables is important for good health. Most of us are
guilty of eating our favorite two or three, but unfortunately, we
need a diverse selection to work synergistically in our body
to neutralize all the different types of free radicals. Fruits and
vegetables give us the antioxidant protection that we need,
more now than ever. Cells make up who we are, and they
reproduce by the billions each day.

We are exposed to many free radicals through our
environment. Free radicals give us disease. Free radicals
cause DNA damage. DNA is the little part of the cell that tells

the rest of the cell what to do. Our best defense is to massively increase the antioxidant network because antioxidants eat free radicals. Certain antioxidants protect our brain; others protect our heart, etc. Antioxidants act as a network, not individually. Studies have shown that if you are taking Vitamin E and you have a high level of free radicals, that lone vitamin becomes oxidized itself, and then, it too becomes a free radical. That is why a network of antioxidants is needed to neutralize the different types of free radicals.

Your body has inborn antioxidant enzymes, but these enzymes decrease in activity as we get older. Then, if we develop disease, these healthy enzymes decrease further, and the toxins significantly increase their activity. Dr. Bruce Aimes, Ph.D. states, "You might just as well stand unprotected in front of an x-ray machine as to not get enough fruits and vegetables. The damage to our cells is the same."

The bottom line is simply this: We are what we eat. We cannot make good cells without eating foods with the right nutrients. As we age, and we continue to eat toxic foods, it is impossible to make healthy cells. We need to change our lifestyles and diets and truly think about what we are eating so we can get the necessary nutrients to live a healthy, disease-free life.

ANTI-CANCER AND ANTI-CARDIOVASCULAR NUTRIENTS THAT COMPLIMENT BIOIDENTICAL HORMONES:

Scientists have identified compounds in cruciferous vegetables (broccoli, cauliflower, and kale, are just a few) that specifically neutralize dangerous breakdown products of estrogen that promote breast cancer growth. They also support our liver, which in turn neutralizes the dangerous carcinogenic chemicals we are exposed to every day. These compounds have a favorable effect on estrogen metabolism and cell division, helping to rid the body of excess estrogen. Cruciferous vegetables play a very important part in maintaining healthy hormone levels.

Cruciferous vegetables are also high in fiber. Other foods that are high in fiber are avocados, artichokes, raspberries, blackberries, black beans, pears, and apples, to name a few. The depletion of vitamins and minerals in the soil and the presence of pesticides and fertilizers create an environment of estrogen dominance. Fiber binds up, deactivates, and excretes excess estrogen and carcinogenic chemicals from the body. The lack of fiber in our diet is connected to many cancers such as colon, breast, lymph, and prostate. Low fiber is also related to heart disease and diabetes. Studies have shown that we need 25-35 grams of fiber a day. Most of us eat about 5 grams.

Eating whole food is the answer to disease prevention. It is an overall consensus worldwide that fruits and vegetables not only reduce the rate of cancer but also prevent atherosclerosis and heart disease. Fruits and vegetables are life-saving foods, but we need more than just a couple, we need a variety without pesticides, herbicides, and poor soil. At least 150 studies around the world have shown that people who eat the most fruits and vegetable are half as likely to have cancer as those who eat the least.

We have come to a time when we should question what the produce in our supermarkets is subjected to. As Suzanne Somers reminds us, produce is picked before it is ripe and stored for long periods of time. Harmful methods are used to ripen or color it artificially for presentation in the "fresh" produce section. Many of the fruits and vegetables have lost nearly all of their vitamin and mineral content by the time you are in the checkout line. So it makes sense to supplement our daily diet with a whole food product, so we are assured of getting the necessary vegetables, fruits, and fiber that we need for a healthy diet, which in turn compliments the best way to achieve a healthy and balanced hormonal system.

I hope this information gives you the confidence to search out a knowledgeable practitioner who will listen and honor your choices, and to share with you a partnership so that you can reclaim your health and well-being. I have been researching bioidentical hormones for more than 20 years. This has become a passion for me. As I see wonderful changes within myself and my clients, I am convinced that hormonal balance is a positive way to help make the rest of your journey healthy and disease-free for a very long time. Keep in mind, each of us is an individual. Individualization in hormone balancing is a necessity. Knowledge is power! Understanding how things work is a great advantage to getting quality care. I hope this informative book will inspire, empower, and equip you with the knowledge necessary so you can have a partnership with your doctor to work together as a team so you can live a more natural, purposeful, and passion-filled life. The power is within all of us to take responsibility for our health!

RESOURCES

HORMONE TESTING:

ZRT Laboratory
12505 NW Cornell Rd.
Portland, OR 97213
www.zrtlab.com
503-469-0741

Genova Diagnostic Laboratory
63 Zillicoa St.
Asheville, NC 28801
www.GDX.net
800-522-4762

COMPOUNDING PHARMACIES:

Pharm.a.care
Florala Pharmacy
1314 E. Fifth Ave.
Florala, Al 36442
Floralapharmacy.com
pharmacare@cyou.com
800-423-7847
Fax 334-858-3550
Tom Frye, P.D. (compounding pharmacist)—Tom has been my personal pharmacist, as well as my dear friend. He

has exceptional knowledge of bioidentical hormones and welcomes your phone calls. He could be your personal pharmacist, too. He offers mail order prescriptions.

International Academy of Compounding Pharmacists (IACP)
P.O. Box 1365
Sugar Land, TX 77487
800-927-4227
Fax: 281-495-0602
www.iacprx.org
This organization has over 1,000 members and will provide the name of a compounding pharmacy in your city.

Compounding Pharmacy of Green
Charles W. Cather, RPh, MBA, FASCP
4016 Massillon Rd., Suite B
Uniontown, Ohio 44685
1-866-797-2667
Fax: 330-899-0652
http://greencompounding.com
Email *cwpharm@hotmail.com*
Charles Cather is an expert in the field of bioidentical hormones, and he would be happy to be your personal pharmacist. He is genuinely interested in the health of his patients. He will work with you and your doctor so you can maintain hormone balance. For your convenience, mail order is available.

Med Quest Compounding Pharmacy Online
Compounding pharmacy and doctor reference
www.mqrx.com

Compounding Pharmacy of Green
Rosario Carcione, Pharm D
4016 Massillon Rd., Suite B

Uniontown, Oh 44685
330-899-0406

RC Compounding
3030 Center Rd.
Poland, Oh 44514
330-707-9001
http://rccompounding.com

DOCTOR REFERRALS:

Natural Woman's Institute (NWI)
8539 Sunset Blvd, #135
Los Angeles, CA 90069
http://instituteofwomanshealth.com
There is knowledge here for practitioners as well as women
wanting to achieve their optimal health.

American Academy of Anti-Aging Medicine (A4M)
1341 W. Fullerton, Suite 111
Chicago, IL 60614
773-528-4333

American College for Advancement in Medicine (ACAM)
8001 Irvine Center Drive, Suite 825
Irvine, California 92618
888-439-6891 or 800-532-3688
www.acam.org
This nonprofit healthcare practitioner organization can help you
find professionals who specialize in an integrative approach to
wellness, including natural/bioidentical hormones.

American Holistic Medical Association (AHMA)
27629 Chagrin Blvd., Suite 213
Woodmere, OH 44122
216-292-6644
This nonprofit healthcare practitioner organization can help you find professionals who specialize in a holistic/integrative approach to wellness, including natural/bioidentical hormones.

Fedorko Chiropractic Health Center
4774 Munson Street NW, Suite 302
Canton, OH 44718
330-497-0422
www.fedorkohealth.com
drfedorko@fedorkohealth.com
I have been a patient of Dr. Fedorko D.C. for 20+ years. He is not only a kinesiologist/chiropractor; he is extremely knowledgeable about nutrition and lab work. He could make a difference in your life. He has a 5-star rating.

Emley Family Chiropractic, Inc.
387 Edgebrook Blvd.
Bolivar, OH 44612
330-874-3542
http://emleychiropratic.com
Dr. Emley is a trusting, personal, and caring chiropractor/kinesiologist. Nutrition plays a key role in his practice. He has a 5-star rating.

International College of Integrative Medicine (ICIM)
Box 271
Bluffton, OH 45817
This nonprofit physician organization can help you find doctors who treat patients with natural/bioidentical hormones.
www.icimed.com
419- 358-0273

Joel Yaffa, M.D.
www.PersonalHormones.com
dryaffa@personalhormones.com
Skype: dryaffa
845-943-2051
Fax: 845-618-1288

Michael E. Greer, M.D.
Holistic, Herbal, Homeopathic Lectures & Consultations
737 Olive Way, #1804
Seattle, WA 98101-3744
michaelgreermd@gmail.com
www.michaelgreermd.com
Cell: 425-243-9308
Fax: 206-971-7428

Dr. Nancy Fazekus Grubb, M.D., ABFM, ABIHM
4030 Massillon Rd., Ste C
Uniontown, OH 44685
office@optimalhealthinstitueohio.com
330-699-1500
330-699-1646
A patient-centered and holistic approach to wellness. Dr. Nancy has been my bioidentical hormone specialist for many years now. She not only balances your hormones, but she also treats the underlying causes of illness, not just symptoms.

WEBSITES FOR BIOIDENTICAL HORMONE RESEARCH:

Dr. Rebecca L. Glaser M.D., FACS
milleniumwellness@gmail.com
www.hormonebalance.org

This site offers 1600 peer-reviewed research studies on the topics of bioidentical hormone replacement. If you go into the data research site of Dr. Rebecca L. Glaser M.D., FACS, you will need to use the word "data" for your user word and "data" for your password.

What's Wilson's Temperature Syndrome?
Dr. James Wilson M.D. coined the term "ADRENAL FATIGUE" in those who had symptoms of suboptimal adrenal function.
www.wilsonssyndrome.com
www.adrenalfatigue.org

Nutrition &Healing
Dr. Glenn S. Rothfeld, M.D.
www.nutritionandhealing.com

Virginia Hopkins News Watch
www.healthwatch@virginiahopkinshealthwatch.com
This is a free newsletter with up-to-date information on natural hormones.

Program in Integrative Medicine/scroll down to Jeanne Drisko M.D.
www.integrativemed.kumc.edu

Dr. Erika Schwartz, M.D.
Dr. Schwartz is a patient health advocate and leading expert on bioidentical hormones
www.drerika.com and *https://eshealth.com*

Dr. Michael Lam, M.D., M.P.H., A.B.A.A.M.
Dr. Lam will help guide you with step-by-step strategies to help with adrenal recovery.
www.DrLam.com

REFERENCES

CHAPTER 1: SYNTHETIC HORMONES VERSUS BIOIDENTICAL HORMONES

Conrad, Christine. *A Woman's Guide to Natural Hormones: For Every Age For Every Stage.* New York, NY: The Berkley Publishing Group/Penguin Group, 2005; 3-13, 64, 69.

Hotze, Steven F. M.D. *Hormones, Health, and Happiness.* Houston, TX: Forrest Publishing, 2005; 111-112.

Lee, John R., M.D. *What Your Doctor May Not Tell You About MENOPAUSE: The Breakthrough Book on Natural Hormone Balance.* New York, NY: Time Warner Book Group, 1996; 31, 69, 130-131.

National Institute of Environmental Health Sciences. "New Federal Report on Carcinogens" Lists Estrogen Therapy. Dec. 11, 2002. *http://www.nih.gov/news/pr/dec2002/niehs-11.htm.*

NHLBI 2002, "NHLBI Stops Trial of Estrogen Plus Progestin Due to Increased Breast Cancer Risk, Lack of Overall Benefit." (online) available at http://www.nhlbi.nih.gov/news/press-releases/2002/nhlbi-stops-trial-of-estrogen-plus-progestin-due-to-increased-breast-cancer-risk-lack-of-overall-benefit.html.

Northrup, Christiane, M.D. The Wisdom of Menopause Creating Physical and Emotional Health and Healing During The Change. New York, NY: Bantam Dell, 2001; 86.

Randolph, C. W., Jr. M.D. *From Hormone Hell to Hormone Well.* Jacksonville Beach, FL: Natural Hormone Institute of America, Inc. 2004; 6, 24, 79-81, 85.

Reiss, Uzzi, M.D. O.B./GYN. *Natural Hormone Balance for Women Look Younger, Feel Stronger, and Live Life with Exuberance.* New York: Pocket Books, 2001; 210-213.

Rossouw, Jaques, July 9, 2002. "Postmenopausal Hormone Therapy." http://www.nhlbi.nih.gov/health/women/rossouw. htm. (accessed 19 Nov. 2010).

Stronger, and Live Life with Exuberance. New York, NY: Pocket Books, 2001; 10, 23, 28.

WHI 2004, NHLBI "Advisory for Physicians on the WHI Trial of Conjugated Equine Estrogens Versus Placebo." http:// www.nhlbi.nih.gov/whi/e-a_advisory.htm. (accessed 25 Nov. 2010).

WHI 2008, "Hormone Therapy Increases Frequency of Abnormal Mammograms and Breast Biopsies" (online) available at https://cleo.whi.org/participants/findings/ Pages/ht_eplusp_mam.aspx (accessed 19 Nov. 2010).

"Wild Yam" 2011: University of Maryland Medical Center (UMMC). www.umm.edu/altmed/articles/wild-yam-000280.htm.

Wright, Jonathan V. M.D. *Natural Hormone Replacement.* Petaluma, CA: Smart Publications, 1997; 21, 49, 54.

CHAPTER 2: PREGNENOLONE

Lee, John R. M.D. *What Your Doctor May Not Tell You About MENOPAUSE: The Breakthrough Book on Natural Hormone Balance.* New York: Time Warner Book Group, 1996; 326-327.

Reiss, Uzzi, M.D.O.B./GYN. *Natural Hormone Balance for Women: Look Younger, Feel Stronger, and Live Life with Exuberance.* New York: Pocket Books, 2001; 210-213.

Reiss, Uzzi, M.D.O.B./GYN. *The Natural Superwoman: The Scientifically Backed Program for Feeling Great, Looking Younger, and Enjoying Amazing Energy at Any Age.* New York: Penguin Group, 2007; 164-173.

Rouzier, Neil, M.D. FACEP. *How To Achieve Healthy Aging-- Look, Live And Feel Fantastic After 40.* Salt Lake City, UT: WorldLink Medical Publishing, 2001; 42-48.

Verneda Lights. "Pregnenolone Deficiency Symptoms." June 14, 2011: www.livestrong.com/article/268663-pregnenolone-deficiency-symptoms.

CHAPTER 3: ESTROGEN

Conrad, Christine. *A Woman's Guide to Natural Hormones: For Every Age For Every Stage.* New York: Berkley Publishing Group/Penguin Group, 2005; 66. JAMA, Jan. 2 1978, Vol. 239, No. 1, pp. 29-30.

Hotze, Steven F. M.D. *Hormones, Health, and Happiness: A Natural Medical Formula for Rediscovering Youth with*

Bioidentical Hormones. Houston, TX: Forrest Publishing, 2005; 98, 104.

Howard Feirman, BS, R PH: Bioidentical Hormone Replacement Therapy. Prescription Headquarters. *http://linchitzwellness.com/index.php?md=95* (accessed 7 Nov. 2010). JAMA, Jan. 18, 1995, Vol 273, No. 3, pp. 199-208.

Lee, John R. M.D. *Dr. John Lee's Hormone Balance Made Simple The Essential How-to Guide to Symptoms, Dosage, Timing, and More.* New York: Warner Books, 2006; 76-77, 82, 85.

Lee, John R. M.D. *What Your Doctor May Not Tell You About MENOPAUSE: The Breakthrough Book on Natural Hormone Balance.* New York: Time Warner Book Group, 1996; 39, 42-43, 140.

McKenna, Saundra. C.N.M. *The Phytogenic Hormone Solution.* New York: Random House, Inc., 2002; 6-9, 25, 37.

Reiss, Uzzi, M.D. O.B./GYN. *Natural Hormone Balance for Women: Look Younger, Feel Stronger, and Live Life with Exuberance.* New York: Pocket Books, 2001; 28-30, 36-37, 57.

Reiss, Uzzi, M.D. O.B./GYN. *The Natural Superwoman: The Scientifically Backed Program for Feeling Great, Looking Younger, and Enjoying Amazing Energy at Any Age.* New York: Penguin Group, 2007; 75-76, 78.

Wright, Jonathan V. M.D. *Natural Hormone Replacement.* Petaluma, CA: Smart Publications, 1997; 57, 56.

CHAPTER 4: PROGESTERONE

Conrad, Christine. *A Woman's Guide to Natural Hormones: For Every Age For Every Stage.* New York: Berkley Publishing Group/Penguin Group, 2005; 76.

Laux, Marcus and Conrad, Christine. *Natural Women Natural Menopause.* New York, NY: HarperCollins Publishers Inc, 1997; 62-70, 72-76.

Lee, John R M.D. *Dr. John Lee's Hormone Balance Made Simple: The Essential How-to Guide to Symptoms, Dosage, Timing, and More.* New York: Warner Books, 2006; 96-122, 130-135.

Lee, John R. M.D. *What Your Doctor May Not Tell You About MENOPAUSE: The Breakthrough Book on Natural Hormone Balance.* New York: Time Warner Book Group, 1996; 69, 309.

McKenna, Saundra. C.N.M. *The Phytogenic Hormone Solution: Restoring Your Delicate Balance with Compounded Natural Hormones.* New York: Random House, Inc., 2002; 9-10, 23-24, 35-36, 47-49.

Prior, J.C. Endocrine Reviews 1990, Vol. 11:2; 386-398 and Prior et al. Canadian Journal of Obstetrics/Gynecology & Women's Health Care 1991; 3:178-84.

Randolph, C.W. Jr. M.D. *From Hormone Hell to Hormone Well.* Jacksonville Beach, FL: Natural Hormone Institute of America, Inc. 2004; 112-128.

Reiss, Uzzi, M.D. O.B/GYN. *The Natural Superwoman: The Scientifically Backed Program for Feeling Great, Looking Younger, and Enjoying Amazing Energy at Any Age.* New York: Penguin Group, 2007; xii, 99-103, 115-123, 148.

Wright, Jonathan V. M.D. *Natural Hormone Replacement.* Petaluma, CA: Smart Publications, 1997; 67, 72, 101-102, 116.

CHAPTER 5: TESTOSTERONE

Lee, John R. M.D. *Dr. John Lee's Hormone Balance Made Simple The Essential How-to Guide to Symptoms, Dosage, Timing, and More.* New York: Warner Books, 2006; 92-93, 95.

Lee, John R. M.D. *What Your Doctor May Not Tell You About MENOPAUSE: The Breakthrough Book on Natural Hormone Balance.* New York: Time Warner Book Group, 1996; 112 -114, 330.

McKenna, Saundra. C.N.M. *The Phytogenic Hormone Solution.* New York: Random House, Inc., 2002; 27, 38.

Randolph, C. W., Jr. M.D. *From Hormone Hell to Hormone Well.* Jacksonville Beach, FL: Natural Hormone Institute of America, Inc. 2004; 234.

Reiss, Uzzi, M.D. O.B./GYN. *The Natural Superwoman: The Scientifically Backed Program for Feeling Great, Looking Younger, and Enjoying Amazing Energy at Any Age.* New York: Penguin Group, 2007; 175-197.

Reiss, Uzzi, M.D. O.B./GYN. *Natural Hormone Balance for Women: Look Younger, Feel Stronger, and Live Life with Exuberance.* New York: Pocket Books, 2001; 165-175.

Rouzier, Neil, M.D. FACEP. *How To Achieve Healthy Aging: Look, Live And Feel Fantastic After 40.* Salt Lake UT: City, WorldLink Medical Publishing, 2001; 20.

Wright, Jonathan V. M.D. *Natural Hormone Replacement.* Petaluma, CA: Smart Publications, 1997; 84-85.

CHAPTER 6: DHEA

Conrad, Christine. *A Woman's Guide to Natural Hormones/ Bioidentical Hormones for Every Age and Every Stage.* New York: The Berkley Publishing Group/Penguin Group, 2005; 81-82, 145-146.

Lee, John R. M.D. *What Your Doctor May Not Tell You About MENOPAUSE: The Break-through Book on Natural Hormone Balance.* New York: Time Warner Book Group, 1996; 111-112, 325-326.

McKenna, Saundra. C.N.M. *The Phytogenic Hormone Solution.* New York: Random House, Inc., 2002; 26-27, 37-38.

Reiss, Uzzi, M.D./O.B. Gyn. *Natural Hormone Balance for Women: Look Younger, Feel Stronger, and Live Life with Exuberance.* New York, NY: Pocket Books, 2001; 194-202.

Reiss, Uzzi, M.D. O.B./GYN. *The Natural Superwoman: The Scientifically Backed Program for Feeling Great, Looking*

Younger, and Enjoying Amazing Energy at Any Age. New York: Penguin Group, 2007; 144-154, 159, 162.

Rouzier, Neil, M.D. FACEP. How To Achieve Healthy Aging: Look, Live And Feel Fantastic After 40. Salt Lake UT: City, WorldLink Medical Publishing, 2001; 19-22, 25, 35, 37-38.

Wright, Jonathan V. M.D. Natural Hormone Replacement. Petaluma, CA: Smart Publications, 1997; 84-85.

CHAPTER 7: MELATONIN

Kava, R., & Herbert, V. (2016, March 07). The Miracle of Melatonin? Retrieved from https://www.acsh.org/news/1995/10/01/the-miracle-of-melatonin.

"Melatonin and Sleep Problems." Melatonin and sleep problems, 2/19/2006. <http//www.webmd.com/hw/health_guide_atoz/aa1863.asp.

Melatonin?>Health Issues> ACSH. Oct.1,1995.11/20/2010. www.acsh.org/healthissues/newsID.747/healthissues_detail.asp.

"Melatonin," The Future in Fitness Certification, 2004. http://www.aftacertification.com/melatonin.htm.

Reiss, Uzzi, M.D./O.B.GYN. Natural Hormone Balance for Women: Look Younger, Fee l Stronger, and Live Life with Exuberance. New York, NY: Pocket Books, 2001; 204-209.

Reiss, Uzzi, M.D., O.B./GYN. The Natural Superwoman: The Scientifically Backed Program for Feeling Great, Looking

Younger, and Amazing Energy at Any Age. New York, NY: Penguin Group, 2007; 283-289.

Rouzier, Neil, M.D. FACEP. *How To Achieve Healthy Aging: Look, Live And Feel Fantastic After 40.* Salt Lake City, UT: WorldLink Medical Publishing, 2001; 50-51, 56-62.

*Slagel, Priscilla, M.D. "Are you shuffling or tap dancing Through life ...or???." The Way Up Newsletter Vol. 7, 1999. 1/16/2011.*www.thewayup.com/newsletters/041599.htm.

Somers, Suzanne. *Ageless: The Naked Truth about Bioidentical Hormones.* New York, NY: Crown Publishing, 2006; 61-64.

"What is Melatonin?" 6/14/2017. *http://www.webmd.com/ sleep-disorders/what-is-melatonin.* Accessed 4/8/2018.

CHAPTER 8: THYROID

Brownstein, David. *Iodine: Why You Need It, Why You Can't Live Without It* 2nd ed. West Bloomfield, MI Medical Alternatives Press, 2006; 19, 25-26, 28, 94, 129-131, 134.

Hotze, Steven F. M.D. *Hormones, Health, and Happiness.* Houston, TX: Forrest Publishing, 2005; 66-84.

Lee, John R. M.D. *What Your Doctor May Not Tell You About MENOPAUSE*: The Breakthrough Book on Natural Hormone Balance. New York: Time Warner Book Group, 1996; 271-273.

Manner, M.G., et al. Salt Iodization for the Elimination of Iodine Deficiency. International Council for the Control of Iodine Deficiency Disorders. 1995.

McKenna, Saundra. C.N.M. *The Phytogenic Hormone Solution*. New York, NY: Random House, Inc., 2002; 28-31, 38-39.

Rouzier, Neil, M.D. FACEP. *How To Achieve Healthy Aging: Look, Live And Feel Fantastic After 40*. Salt Lake City, UT: WorldLink Medical Publishing, 2001; 153-179.

Shames, Richard L. M.D. *Thyroid Power: 10 Steps To Total Health*. New York, NY: Harper Collins Publishers Inc., 2002.

Somers, Suzanne. *Ageless: The Naked Truth about Bioidentical Hormones*. New York, NY: Crown Publishing, 2006; 44-47.

Somers, Suzanne. *Breakthrough: Eight Steps to Wellness*. New York, NY: Crown Publishing, 2008; 120-122, 133-134.

CHAPTER 9: IODINE AND THYROID FUNCTION

Ageless: The Naked Truth about Bioidentical Hormones. New York, NY: Crown Publishing, 2006; 210-211, 365.

Brownstein, David. *Iodine: Why You Need It, Why You Can't Live Without It* 2nd ed. West Bloomfield, MI Medical Alternatives Press, 2006; 19, 25-26, 28, 94, 129, 134.

Heyduk, Danielle, December 1, 2009. "Iodine Deficiency: More Prevalent Than Ever Before." http://www.associatedcontent.

com/article/1674039/iodine_deficiency. (Accessed 19 November 2010).

Reiss, Uzzi, M.D./O.B./GYN. *The Natural Superwoman*. New York, NY: Penguin Group, 2007; 330.

Somers Suzanne. *Breakthrough*. New York, NY: Crown Publishing, 2008, 36-37, 230, 261.

Stadel, B. Dietary iodine and risk of breast, endometrial and ovarian cancer. The Lancet. 4.24. 1976 Dietary iodine and risk of breast cancer. British J. of Cancer. 1997; 75(11):1699-1703.

CHAPTER 10: ADRENAL FUNCTION

Hotze, Steven F. M.D. *Hormones, Health, and Happiness*. Houston, TX: Forrest Publishing, 2005; 136-149.

Jefferies, William McK. M.D. F.A.C.P. *Safe Uses of Cortisol*. Springfield, Ill: Charles C. Thomas Publisher, LTD. 2004.

Lam, Michael, M.D., M.P.H. *Adrenal Fatigue Syndrome Reclaim Your Energy and Vitality with Clinically Proven Natural Programs*. Loma Linda, CA: Adrenal Institute Press, 2012.

Lee, John R. M.D. *What Your Doctor May Not Tell You About MENOPAUSE: The Breakthrough Book on Natural Hormone Balance*. New York, NY: Time Warner Book Group, 1996; 122-123,141-146.

McKenna, Saundra. C.N.M. *The Phytogenic Hormone Solution.* New York, NY: Random House, Inc., 2002; 31-35, 39-40.

Randolph, C. W., Jr. M.D. *From Hormone Hell to Hormone Well.* Jacksonville Beach, FL: Natural Hormone Institute of America, Inc. 2004; 176-184.

Reiss, Uzzi, M.D. O.B./GYN *The Natural Superwoman.* New York, NY: Penguin Group, 2007; 219, 225, 227.

Taylor, Edward, M.D. "The Adrenal Glands." BHRT World Summit. Dr. Joel Yaffa, M.D. 2008; 2.

Wilson, James L. N.D. D. C., Ph.D. *Adrenal Fatigue The 21st Century Stress Syndrome.* Petaluma, CA: Smart Publications, 2001.

Wilson, James, Dr. "Are You Experiencing Adrenal Fatigue?" 2013; *www.adrenalfatigue.org.*

CHAPTER 11: VITAMIN D

Cerhan JR, Sellers TA, Janney CA, et al. Prenatal and perinatal correlates of adult mammographic breast density. *Cancer Epidemiol Biomarkers Prev. 2005 Jun; 4(6):1502-8.*

Franklin GM, Nelson L. Environmental risk factors in multiple sclerosis: causes, triggers, and patient autonomy. *Neurology. 2003 Oct 28; 61(8):1032-4.*

Grant WB, Holick MF. Benefits and requirements of vitamin D for optimal health: a review. *Altern Med Rev. 2005 June; 10(2):94-111.*

Hathcock JN, Shao A., Vieth R., Heaney R. Risk assessment for Vitamin D. *Am J Clin Nutr. 2007; 85:6-18.*

Hypponen E, Laara E, Reunanen A, Jarvelin MR, Virtanen SM. Intake of vitamin D and risk of type I diabetes: a birth-cohort study. *Lancet.* 2001 Nov. 3; 358(9292):1500-3.

Hypponen E. Micronutrients and the risk of type 1 diabetes: vitamin D, vitamin E, and nicotinamide. *Nutr Rev. 2004* Sept; 62(9):340-7. Available at: http//ods.od.nih.gov/factsheets/vitaminD—Quickfacts.asp. November 17, 2005.

John EM, Schwartz GG, Koo J, Van Den BD, Ingles SA. Sun exposure, vitamin D receptor gene polymorphisms, and risk of advanced prostate cancer. *Cancer Res. 2005 Jun 15; 65(12):5470-9.*

Lehmann B. The vitamin D3 pathway in human skin and its role for regulation of biological processes. *Photochem Photobiol.* 2005 Feb.1.

Lou YR Qiao S, Talonpoika R, Syvala H, Tuohimaa P. The role of vitamin D3 metabolism in prostate cancer. *Steroid Biochem Mol Biol.* 2004 Nov; 92(4):317-25.

Wolters M. Diet and psoriasis: experimental data and clinical evidence. Br J Dermatol. 2005 Oct; 153(4):706-14.

Zhou W, Suk R, Liu G, et al. Vitamin D is associated with improved survival in early-stage non-small cell lung cancer patients. *Cancer Epidemiol Biomarkers Prev. 2005 Oct; 14(10):2303-9.*

CHAPTER 12: TESTS TO DO BEFORE BEGINNING BIOIDENTICAL HORMONES

Reiss, Uzzi, M.D./O.B. Gyn. *Natural Hormone Balance for Women: Look Younger, Feel Stronger, and Live Life with Exuberance.* New York, NY: Pocket Books, 2001; 38-40, 77-78.

Somers, Suzanne. *Breakthrough: Eight Steps to Wellness.* New York, NY: Crown Publishing, 2008; 56-57,198-199.

CHAPTER 14: CANCER, DIET, AND BIOIDENTICAL HORMONES

Dr. Richard DuBois. The Whole Truth in 15 Minutes. www.withaweb.com/wholetruth.htm (accessed Sept. 1-Nov. 8, 2010).

From an interview with Dr. John Potter in *Nutrition Action Health Letter,* April 1994, published by the Center for Science in the Public Interest.

Jemal, Ahmedin DVM, Ph.D., Rebecca Siegel, MPH, Xu Jiaquan M.D., and Ward, Elizabeth PhD, "Cancer Statistics," 2010: CA Cancer J Clin 2010. doi:10.3322/caac.20073.

Somers, Suzanne. *Breakthrough: Eight Steps to Wellness.* New York: Crown Publishing, 2008; 88, 186-187, 200-201, 315-317.

Silverberg, Edwin & Grant, Roald N., "A Cancer Journal for Clinicians" (1970; 20; 10-230). www.caonline. amcancersoc.org/cgi/reprint/20/1/10.pdf.

Taylor, Elder B. M.D. *Are your hormones making you sick?* Orem, UT: Abridged Version Published, 2004; 142-186.

INDIVIDUAL HORMONE CONSULT

sue.berkey@gmail.com

KNOWLEDGE IS POWER

- I can help you navigate through the maze of BHRT on a personal level.
- Do you want help finding a knowledgeable doctor and compounding pharmacy near you?
- I will help direct you and give you the necessary guidance for your individual needs.
- If expense is an issue, I can teach you how to have your compounding pharmacist help you with the guidance of your family doctor.

IT IS IMPORTANT FOR YOU TO BE AN INFORMED PATIENT!

Note from the Publisher

Are you a first time author?

Not sure how to proceed to get your book published?
Want to keep all your rights and all your royalties?
Want it to look as good as a Top 10 publisher?
Need help with editing, layout, cover design?
Want it out there selling in 90 days or less?

Visit our website for some exciting new options!

Manufactured by Amazon.ca
Bolton, ON

18510716R00061